COPING WITH CHRONIC FATIGUE

·TRUDIE CHALDER is a lecturer in the Department of Psychological Medicine, King's College Hospital and the Institute of Psychiatry, London. She has worked extensively with individuals with chronic fatigue syndrome and has been researching into the causes and treatment of fatigue over the past seven years. Her work has been published in a number of academic journals. While writing this book she was supported by the Linbury Trust.

Overcoming Common Problems

COPING WITH CHRONIC FATIGUE

Trudie Chalder

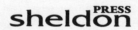

First published in Great Britain in 1995 by
Sheldon Press, SPCK, Marylebone Road, London NW1 4DU

Fifth impression 2000

British Library Cataloguing-in-Publication Data
A catalogue record for this book is available from the British Library

ISBN 0-85969-685-5

Photoset by Deltatype Ltd, Ellesmere Port, Cheshire
Printed in Great Britain by Biddles Ltd, *www.biddles.co.uk*

Contents

To Nora Spring

Acknowledgements

First and foremost I would like to thank an ex-colleague and friend Sue Butler who helped pioneer the treatment approach described in this book. Second, and most importantly, I am appreciative of the feedback I have received from patients with chronic fatigue whom I have treated using the approach described in this book. They have been an endless source of encouragement to me in my work. Despite tremendous disabilities, they have shown how a collaborative venture can enable them to lead active and fulfilling lives once again.

Preface

Chronic fatigue has always been a problem for doctors. It is one of the commonest symptoms encountered in the community – a recent survey found that 30 per cent of women and 20 per cent of men admitted to always feeling tired for every day during the previous month. Doctors tend to prefer the recherché and unusual to the common or garden problems of everyday life. Chronic fatigue does not kill, and hence is not accompanied by the drama beloved of medical students and viewers of *Casualty*. It is also non-specific: coughing up blood or crushing central chest pain have a limited number of causes, well known to doctors, but chronic fatigue could be a symptom of virtually any disease, physical or psychological. In consequence, chronic fatigue occupies little space in medical textbooks or curricula.

During the last few years there have been signs of a change, for two reasons. The first has been a series of studies carried out in the community and general practice. These have shown that although chronic fatigue is both common and non fatal, it is certainly not a trivial complaint. Studies have shown that chronically fatigued patients encounter difficulties in many aspects of their lives, with dramatic effects on their ability to work and look after homes and families.

The second has been the appearance of a new disease, variously called chronic fatigue syndrome (CFS), myalgic encephalomyelitis (ME) or post-viral fatigue syndrome. CFS is not actually a new disease, but there can be no doubt that it has caught the attention of both media and public alike. Exactly what causes it is far from certain. It has been claimed to be due to a viral infection, a disturbance of muscles, an immune dysfunction or a biochemical disorder of the brain. It has also been claimed to be psychological, linked to depression or anxiety. Finally some sceptics say it doesn't exist at all.

It now seems very unlikely to be due to a single virus, or to be a muscle disease. Psychological problems are certainly common, but their cause is still unclear. Instead, most experts now agree that CFS or ME is unlikely to be one disease, but probably a variety of conditions. It also almost certainly has more than one cause, in the same way that heart disease is the end point of a number of factors, such as genetics, smoking, stress, diet and poor exercise. We have also argued that CFS may not be a discrete condition at all, but represents the end of a spectrum of fatigue and exhaustion, in the same way that very high blood pressure represents the dangerous end of the spectrum of blood pressure, starting with normal values.

Although the arrival of CFS or ME has generated a considerable amount of heat, it has not always generated much light. The often intense controversy surrounding the subject shows us that our pious hopes that psychological distress is treated as seriously as physical illness is just that – a pious hope – as, instead, professionals and the media continue to be drawn into futile arguments about whether the problem is physical or psychological. One consequence has been the neglect of perhaps the most important aspect of chronic fatigue and chronic fatigue syndrome – what to do about it.

The medical and professional literature is almost silent on the subject of treatment, instead concentrating on issues such as immunology, virology or psychiatry, none of which can yet help sufferers. There have been several popular books on the subject, but none have combined a coherent, scientific knowledge of the subject with a practical, pragmatic approach to management.

It is thus a great pleasure to write this introduction to Trudie Chalder's book. In the following pages Ms Chalder provides a succinct review of the subject, and then provides a sensible approach to the self-management of chronic fatigue. Behind her approach is a style of rehabilitation known as cognitive behaviour therapy. This sounds rather technical, but is actually a very pragmatic and common-sense approach to recovery. It has been widely used in a number of illnesses, ranging from the physical to the psychological, but has been particularly valuable in the treatment of another condition which has a great deal of overlap with chronic fatigue, and also involves a mixture of physical and psychological factors – chronic pain.

Cognitive behaviour therapy is not new. However, Trudie Chalder has played the major role in adapting it for the particular problems of the sufferer from chronic fatigue or chronic fatigue syndrome. Since she started this pioneering work many others have followed, and it is rapidly becoming the mainstay of treatment offered by a number of teams around the world. It is not, of course, the answer to all the problems of chronic fatigue, but it is certainly a practical, useful and effective approach.

Trudie has taught me most of what I know about treating chronically fatigued patients, and thus I am delighted she has now written a straightforward account for non-professionals.

Simon Wessely
King's College, London

Introduction

'Tired', 'exhausted', 'weak', 'drained', 'lethargic' – these are all words you may have used to describe the feeling of fatigue. Feeling tired is usually a signal from your body that you need to rest – so not everyone who feels tired is ill. Some people with fatigue feel very tired all of the time but are able to do most things in spite of it. Others are so incapacitated by fatigue they are unable to carry on with their everyday lives. Feeling tired is so common we consider it normal. In order to avoid confusion, in this book, we will consider fatigue to be an illness if the person finds it necessary to seek help.

You may have been told, and believe, there is nothing you can do about fatigue. However, once you have accepted that fatigue is a real problem for you, this book can help you, step by step, to draw on all your resources to regain control of your life.

The first step is to understand fatigue, which, like many health issues, is a complicated one. The second step is to look at how your thoughts and actions influence how you feel. The third step is to develop practical ways of coping with and changing fatigue – you will be amazed at how powerful you can become in making positive changes in your life. Finally, you will learn how to cope with difficulties and setbacks.

It is important to understand that it takes months and sometimes years to develop long-term fatigue; it will certainly take many months to overcome it. The process is not an easy one; at times making some of the changes I suggest will seem impossible. However, having worked for many years with people who have had severe and long-

1

term fatigue, I can honestly say that it *is* possible. The very fact that you are reading this book shows you are determined – no matter how tired you may feel at the moment! – to overcome the problem of fatigue.

1
What is fatigue?

Despite being a very common problem, we know very little about fatigue. We do know that it affects more women than men, but it does not seem to affect a particular age group. Nearly everyone feels tired at some time, but only a small proportion of the population feels very tired all of the time.

Some physical illnesses – such as thyroid disease, anaemia, and liver disease – can cause fatigue. Sometimes people develop fatigue after common infections. It can also be a symptom of emotional distress, such as anxiety or depression due to problems at work or home. However, when you visit your doctor, he or she will probably not be able to give you a single, specific explanation as to why you feel so tired all of the time.

When to see your doctor

Everyone experiences physical symptoms such as fatigue, headaches and back pain. At first it may be reasonable to ignore them. However, if the symptom persists, *do take the symptom seriously*. For a few people, severe tiredness can have a physical cause, so it is worth discussing with your doctor the possibility of carrying out routine blood tests. It must be remembered, however, that your tiredness probably will be linked to more than one factor – for example, someone who feels stressed because of worries at home, but also has a physical problem.

Your tiredness could be linked to a psychological illness. Your doctor should be able to help you by assessing whether your symptoms are related to anxiety or depression. If you are depressed, you may be prescribed antidepressants. Alternatively, you may be asked to see a psychiatrist for further assessment, or a counsellor or psychotherapist.

Drugs

Many drugs list fatigue, lethargy, sedation and drowsiness as possible side-effects. Most people who do experience fatigue as a result of taking such drugs find ways of coping. Others have to weigh up whether the benefits outweigh the fatigue.

If you have to take medication for a long-term illness, plan your life according to the effects of the medication. However, before accepting fatigue as a side-effect, check with your doctor if, first, you really need to take the drug, and, second, whether there are any alternatives. If you do have to take medication, you must find a way of dealing with the fatigue. This book should be of help.

Be sure you are taking the correct dose at the right times. If possible, take sedating drugs at night. *Always check with your doctor before changing anything*. If you are taking more than one drug, ask your doctor whether their interaction will affect you.

Chronic fatigue syndrome

If your doctor cannot find an explanation for your tired-ness, he or she may tell you that you have chronic (long-lasting) fatigue syndrome (CFS). This is a good term to use because it is purely descriptive – it does not define the cause of your problem.

Although it has only recently been publicized in the media, in the medical world CFS has been around for a long time – the only difference is that the label has changed. At the end of the last century there was a condition known

4

as neurasthenia with similar symptoms, and before then physicians often diagnosed exhaustion found in soldiers as being due to the stress of battle, described as effort syndrome. During World War One 60,000 British soldiers were diagnosed as having the syndrome, and 44,000 of these were retired because they could no longer function in combat.

In 1934 an American physician suggested that chronic fatigue was caused by a bacterial infection transmitted through farm animals. In the same year there was an outbreak of a strange illness in which patients experienced muscle pain and problems with thinking.

During the last 20 years or so a variety of factors have been associated with CFS, including low blood sugar, candida, several viruses, and allergies. There is no clear-cut evidence that any of these is the primary cause of the syndrome, and it seems more likely that a variety of factors contribute to its development.

Fatigue is a symptom which everyone experiences at some time or another to a lesser or greater extent. The longer the fatigue is present, the greater its severity, the larger the number of associated symptoms, and the greater the degree to which a person's life is affected, the more likely it is that the fatigue will be considered abnormal.

Have you got it?

There is no definitive test for CFS. If you are told this is what you have, your doctor will have based his or her diagnosis on the following. That:

- fatigue is the principal symptom;
- it had a definite onset, and it is not life-long;
- it is severe, disabling, and affects physical and mental functioning;
- it has been present for a minimum of six months, and for more than 50 per cent of the time;

5

- other symptoms may be present, such as muscle pain or sleep and mood disturbance.

CFS does not include people suffering from medical or psychiatric conditions such as anaemia, schizophrenia, manic-depressive illness, drug abuse, eating disorders, or organic brain disease, all of which can cause fatigue.

If you have CFS you probably will say that the kind of tiredness you experience is very different from the normal tiredness you used to feel when you were well. For example, it is often severe and affects both your physical and mental functioning. It also fluctuates: you may feel almost normal and then suddenly feel exhausted again.

Problems with sleep are common: you may not be able to fall asleep, and when you do, you may wake frequently during the night. Or you may be sleeping too much, sometimes up to several hours more than you would have before you became ill. Whatever your complaint, it is likely that sleep is seldom refreshing, and you often wake feeling exhausted.

Your fatigue may be associated with a variety of symptoms, some physical and some mental. Physical symptoms include headaches, dizziness, nausea, tingling in the fingers, shakiness, muscle and joint pain and many others. Or you may have frequent sore throats and infections, which could be a consequence of being run down. Mental symptoms may include concentration difficulties, memory problems and not being able to find the right words.

The mind-body problem

You may feel that your fatigue has not been taken seriously, particularly if your doctor has not been able to detect a recognized physical cause. You may have been told there is nothing wrong with you, and that it is all in your mind. Your problem then becomes either psychological – and therefore not important – or it is just a figment of your imagination. Even if nothing physical can be found it does not mean there is nothing wrong. Physical and psychological causes of fatigue are equally important, and usually something can be done about both.

The power of the mind to influence the body has been recognized for thousands of years. We know that there is a close relationship between the immune system and the brain, and when one system is not working well it will affect the other. This is a perfect example of how the body is inseparable from the mind, and vice-versa.

However, we all get caught in the mind-body trap, saying that a symptom has *either* a psychological *or* a physical cause. It is very common to create an artificial divide between our minds and our bodies. For example, there is no word in the English language which means both mind and body. And yet they are interdependent.

Health professionals are often reluctant to acknowledge the role that our thoughts and emotions play in the state of our health and illness. In fact, everything from the common cold to cancer can be affected by our moods, personalities, attitudes and so on. You probably have experienced this yourself – for example, you may have noticed that if you have been feeling under pressure, you are more likely to catch a cold or have an accident.

In most cases it is unhelpful if you have CFS to continue to search for a single physical cause. Once routine tests have been carried out and your doctor is reassured that further tests would not be helpful, it is more useful for you to think about how your fatigue can be managed.

It is likely that a combination of factors cause fatigue. Some of these are described below. It is not an exhaustive list, but perhaps you will recognize some of them, and how they are important to you.

Are you over-stressed?

You would probably agree that the harder you work, the more stressed you become, the more likely you are to feel fatigued. Unemployment or job-related conflicts, relationship or family difficulties are also some issues that contribute to feeling stressed and, ultimately, fatigued.

Stressful life events such as a death in the family, job change, relationship breakup or changes in the family – even a much-welcomed new baby – are known to contribute to the onset and continuation of chronic fatigue. Stress also can affect the body's immune system, making you more vulnerable to common infections.

You may have tried to cope with your problems by doing things that in the long term will make them worse. For example, if you are a woman, you may be using over- or under-eating to reduce tension. Or you may be smoking or drinking too much. These are common attempts to cope with stress that cause fatigue and other more serious health problems. Drugs of all kinds – sometimes even those prescribed to help – can make your problem worse.

In a life crisis?

There are periods of change in all of our lives that increase our vulnerability. These turning-points usually occur when adjustments and changes have to be made. For example, you may until recently have been dedicated to your career, but discover you now long for marriage and children; or if you are a housewife or mother, you may be itching to start a new career, or return to an old one.

Sometime between their late 30s and 40s, some people

begin to go through the mid-life crisis. They may realize they are not going to live forever, and that the goals and ambitions they had set for themselves may not be achieved. They may also realize they have neglected important areas of their lives – close relationships, creativity, hobbies. Thinking and worrying about such things can bring on depression, stress – and fatigue.

The search for perfection

The desire to do well often turns into a desire to do things perfectly. As there is no such thing as perfection, striving to achieve the impossible usually results in disappointment. Sometimes the drive to succeed is so great that it can prevent you from achieving anything at all. It also can result in anxiety, fatigue and unhappiness.

In today's society people are rewarded for their achievements – success has become a top priority. Doing well and being productive can be rewarding and enjoyable, however, success is not synonymous with happiness, and always striving for better things can lead to low self-esteem and depression.

Having high expectations of yourself has an effect on how much energy you have. You may believe you should not get tired, and if you do there must be something wrong. You may think you don't have as much energy as you used to have, and that you would like to feel like you did five years ago. What you have not taken into account, however, is that you probably have far more responsibilities and stresses in your life now and are bound to feel more tired.

Children have endless amounts of energy, but it is easy to forget that they have no commitments or responsibilities. As adults we often feel we should be able to keep going just as we did when we were children. Throughout our lives we may take on more and more responsibilities at work or at home, without considering the effect this has on our health.

Physical causes of fatigue

One of the contributing factors to your fatigue may have a physical basis. For example, you may have had a viral illness. It may have been a cold, influenza, diarrhoea, vomiting or some other infection. You may have experienced symptoms like tiredness, painful muscles, exhaustion and sweating. Almost certainly you did not feel like doing anything, and may have taken time off work or spent some time in bed. This was a sensible thing to do: vigorous exercise would have been harmful, and rest was needed to help your body combat the infection.

It takes some people longer than others to get over infections. However, nearly everyone recovers completely, and by three months most people are back to what they would call normal.

For some people – perhaps for you – it is not that simple. You may continue to feel unusually tired six months after having had a simple infection. Instead of returning to health, you find yourself trapped in a vicious circle of fatigue, trying to cope and make sense of it, followed by more fatigue.

If your fatigue has continued long after the onset of the initial illness, you may be worried that you still have an infection. There is little evidence of this, or that viruses alone can cause chronic fatigue. Even though a virus may have contributed to your feelings of fatigue in the first place, many other factors play a part in the ongoing problem. Whatever triggered your fatigue in the first place may not be what is keeping it going.

If you experience muscle pain you may worry about whether there is something wrong with your muscles. There is no evidence of this. Muscle function is normal in people with chronic fatigue; the muscles are capable of working normally, even if it does not feel like they are.

If you are an athlete or physically fit you are more likely to experience muscle fatigue and pain. During a period of forced inactivity, your muscles contract. On restarting exercise, especially if you return to high levels of exercise too soon, the muscles are stretched or lengthened. This puts a strain on the muscle, temporarily damages it and causes pain. Strange though it may seem, physically fit people are also more likely to develop infections than unfit individuals. This is probably because they are more sensitive to subtle physical changes occurring to their bodies, and therefore are more likely to respond to them by becoming ill.

Emotional causes of fatigue

All of us have experienced depression at some time or another, in varying degrees. You are probably familiar with the symptoms: lack of energy and motivation, tiredness, an inability to enjoy life, tearfulness; the future may seem hopeless; or you may have a low opinion of yourself, sleep difficulties, poor concentration, loss of appetite, irritability, or loss of sexual interest.

People sometimes develop depression in response to life events. Some people inherit a susceptibility to depression, while others appear to become depressed for no apparent reason. Long-standing difficulties such as relationship problems or long-term unemployment can result in a sense of helplessness that leads to depression.

Feeling helpless and demoralized is an understandable part of chronic illness, and doctors and other health professionals may identify this as depression. As a fatigue sufferer you may feel that a diagnosis of depression suggests that your fatigue is not real. This is not the case.

Whatever the cause, depression is a very real illness for which there are effective physical and psychological treatments.

Frustration is another common reaction to the cycle of symptoms and restrictions imposed by fatigue. You are also likely to feel anxious if you think you should be doing more but at the same time fear an increase in your symptoms. This can become a self-perpetuating and difficult trap to get out of: the more activities you avoid, the more anxious you are likely to become at the thought of trying to do things. Sometimes anxiety and frustration can push you into doing too much too quickly, and sometimes they can stop you from doing anything at all. Fatigue is a symptom of anxiety, and anxiety brings about fatigue.

Activity or rest?

You may think that if you rest in response to feeling tired you will get better and feel rejuvenated. Usually this is the case. However, sometimes you continue to feel tired and the level of your tiredness seems out of proportion to the apparent cause.

How you cope with persistent tiredness depends on a number of factors including personality, advice given by doctors or nurses, individual expectations and past experience. You may rest more in the hope of improvement; or you may exercise vigorously with the aim of beating the problem. Or, you may modify or reduce what you do according to your level of tiredness. Either way, the end result is a see-saw of rest and activity: doing too much one day leads to exhaustion the next; doing nothing for several days leads to feeling even more tired than before.

Are you doing too much?

Many people feel tired for the simple reason that they are

doing too much. Some may be struggling with a difficult job, working long hours and getting insufficient sleep; others are trying to look after a family, run a house and also are not getting enough sleep. Then along comes a viral infection and becomes the 'straw that breaks the camel's back'.

Women in particular struggle to meet the never-ending demands made upon them, tending to meet all of their responsibilities before attending to their own individual needs. They get little sleep, no exercise, and generally have no time for themselves. In addition, they may not receive any recognition for their work and commitment to the family. Many women end up feeling depressed, worn out and too guilty to take any personal time.

Or doing too little?

If you are acutely ill, or when you normally feel tired, you rest to feel better. If you have chronic fatigue, however, the opposite is true. Doing less may help in the short term, but in the long term inactivity makes you feel more exhausted and lethargic:

- Inactivity leads to loss of drive and determination. The less you do, the less you feel like doing, and the harder it feels to do more – even small tasks become daunting.

- Inactivity can make you feel you are losing control of your life and that you are not achieving anything worthwhile; it can deprive you of things that previously gave you pleasure.

- Inactivity may affect your quality of sleep.

- Inactivity reduces physical fitness and muscle strength, and increases muscle fatigue.

13

Excessive rest produces weakness, loss of strength, and fatigue. The fact that many people feel tired because they are doing too much is well known. However, the reverse is equally true – you feel tired because you are doing too little. This might appear to contradict common sense, but it can in fact be understood quite easily.

You may have tried to control your fatigue by reducing what you do, such as spending more time in bed, taking time off work and so on. This is sensible when you are feeling ill. However, if as time goes on, the symptoms of your fatigue persist or get worse, you may avoid or reduce what you do as a way of controlling your symptoms.

Initially you may feel slightly better. However, the next time you do something, your symptoms may recur either immediately or soon after, which seems to confirm that any activity should be avoided or modified. In this way a vicious circle is set in motion: symptoms – avoidance of activity – temporary relief.

As time goes on and you do not feel any better, reducing activity still further results in an increase in your symptoms. So, despite the fact that rest initially lessened your symptoms, the longer-term effects are the opposite – a worsening of symptoms. It is understandable why you might continue to reduce the amount you do because as soon as you attempt to do more your symptoms get worse. However, it is likely that you are doing too much, too soon.

What often happens is that people do both too much and too little. You may alternate periods of doing too much either on days when you feel a little better or in a conscious effort to 'exercise away' your tiredness, with periods of resting in order to recover and to regain your strength. This 'yo-yo' pattern is self-perpetuating, leading to a vicious circle of too much rest, too much exercise, more fatigue and more pain.

The consequences of prolonged rest are a worsening of

symptoms, reduction in activity, feelings of helplessness and demoralization, loss of control and a very restricted life. Doing too little can be as damaging as doing too much.

Negative thinking

Just as what you do influences how you feel, how you think also affects how you feel and what you do. Our thoughts influence our behaviour.

In addition to beliefs about the nature of your illness, you may also have negative thoughts that suddenly pop into your head either before, during or after activity. For example, 'If I do too much today, then tomorrow I'll feel worse.' The effect of such negative thinking is that you may reduce your activity further, which will lead to an increase in symptoms, and to feelings of helplessness and loss of control.

After a period of prolonged ill health it is natural to become more aware of your body. Becoming more aware of symptoms such as fatigue, muscle pain and so on is not always beneficial. You may have noticed that when you think about your fatigue or monitor your symptoms very closely they sometimes get worse. And if you switch your thoughts to something else the symptoms lessen. Although the fatigue does not go away when you are absorbed in something interesting, you notice it less.

On the other hand, you may think it is normal to be constantly 'on the go'. Instead of resting in response to exhaustion, you keep going. You may not have the time to rest very much, but also feel guilty about resting and having some time for yourself. You may feel there is something wrong with you if you are unable to meet all the demands being made upon you without resting. Many people with CFS describe how they used to be energetic, working long hours and going out almost every evening, with little time for relaxation or rest. The only time they rested was when they slept.

If you are like this you may feel that unless you live life in the fast lane you have failed in some way. Negative thoughts are common, for example, 'I should be able to do all the things I used to do. If I can't, then there must be something seriously wrong.' The reason you think such thoughts is because your sense of identity is being threatened: you are what you do; if you do not do enough, you cease to be you.

Conclusion: what causes fatigue

Below is a list of factors which could have influenced your fatigue problem:

- stress, busy lifestyle, little time for enjoyable activities or rest;
- major upheavals or life events such as a job change;
- transition periods;
- perfectionism coupled with high expectations;
- emotional troubles, such as anxiety and depression;
- failure to get over a viral illness;
- coping by either doing too much or too little.

The diagram below shows how physical, emotional and social factors can contribute to the development and maintenance of chronic fatigue.

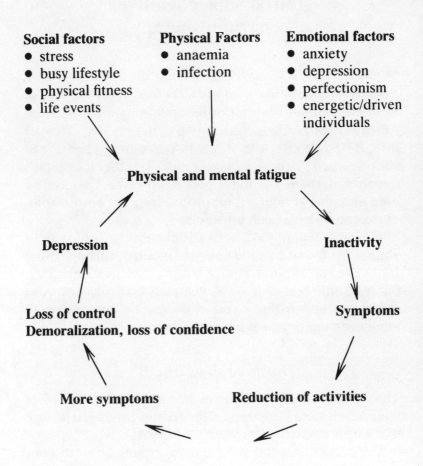

Social factors
- stress
- busy lifestyle
- physical fitness
- life events

Physical Factors
- anaemia
- infection

Emotional factors
- anxiety
- depression
- perfectionism
- energetic/driven individuals

Physical and mental fatigue

Depression

Inactivity

Loss of control
Demoralization, loss of confidence

Symptoms

More symptoms

Reduction of activities

2

Introducing cognitive
behaviour therapy

Cognitive behaviour therapy (CBT) involves the use of specific techniques to alter or modify thoughts and actions which may be working against you getting better. In order for CBT to be effective, it has to be tailored precisely to your needs. For those who are very ill, a therapist works closely with them. For many people however, CBT can be used at home without a therapist, as long as the principles of treatment have been understood.

The idea behind CBT is to strengthen the coping skills you are using that *are* effective, and modify or change those which *are not*. It is not a quick fix. It takes time and effort, but you will find that by developing control over your symptoms and feelings you will develop the ability to influence your personal life and relationships.

The three steps of CBT

The first step in CBT involves keeping a daily record of your activity and symptoms. This creates a detailed picture that forms a baseline for your treatment.

The second step involves a close examination of your activity diaries, focusing on how your symptoms influence how much rest you have or how much you do. Patterns of rest and activity interact with your symptoms, sometimes forming an ever-worsening spiral of disability. One important aspect of CBT is to reverse this spiral by breaking the link between your symptoms and stopping or reducing activity. The emphasis is on consistency. In other words, it is not how much you do, but how *consistently* you do it. Very gradually, step by step, you increase the amount of activity with which you can comfortably cope. With a carefully planned programme of graded, consistent activity and rest it is possible to achieve lasting symptom reduction. If your problem is doing too much, regular rest periods are similarly planned in order to achieve a reduction in fatigue.

The third step involves looking at how your thoughts influence what you are able to do and how you feel. There is a large amount of scientific research that supports the idea that your thoughts or patterns of thinking influence dramatically how you feel and act.

In practice, the doing and thinking aspects of CBT work together. However, to avoid confusion they are discussed separately in the following chapters.

During a CBT programme you will learn that you are able to tolerate symptoms without the same degree of worry as before. While changing your levels of activity, *your symptoms of fatigue will probably get worse before they get better*. However, knowing this will help you to feel less worried about the consequences of your actions and symptoms, and you will start to feel more in control. You will be in charge of your symptoms, rather than them being in control of you. This is because you will understand how your body and mind work together. As time goes on, your confidence will grow and minor setbacks will become less traumatic. This is not always a dramatic change, but slowly you will learn how powerful your thoughts are in influencing how you feel and behave.

How does CBT work?

You probably believe, as most people do, that you should do what your body tells you. This may be true in some situations, such as a 'new' illness, but it is not true in those that are long-standing. Following what your body tells you can cause more harm than good: even though you feel exhausted, rest is not necessarily the way to make yourself feel better.

It is also a popular belief that physical symptoms must have physical causes that can be identified. This is not always the case; symptoms sometimes have clear, identifiable physical causes – but often they do not. Even if symptoms do have an obvious physical cause, they are not always treatable by conventional medical methods.

The effects of inactivity

Why does prolonged inactivity cause your fatigue to get worse rather than better? A reduction in your normal physical activity results in a deconditioning of the neuromuscular system. It impairs the function of your cardiovascular, skeletal and other organ systems.

Your normal muscle strength is maintained by activity – frequent muscle contractions which produce tension. There is a relationship between loss of muscle strength and the ability to carry out activities which require endurance. Strength decreases with bedrest at an average rate of 3 per cent per day. Daily activity is essential.

Clearly, the best way to preserve muscle strength is through normal, daily physical activity. Two to three hours of daily standing and walking seems to prevent problems of disuse. Therefore, a graded, consistent approach to activity, regardless of the cause of your fatigue is essential to prevent loss of your muscle strength.

Just for a moment, let us look at your initial response to a reduction in activity levels – that is, a reduction in fatigue. Experiments have shown that when you do something which is followed by a reward you are likely to do it again. If you reduce activity levels either in response to fatigue or because you fear an increase in symptoms, the symptoms are likely to continue. There is a close connection between your behaviour (reduction in activity), and your response (reduction in fatigue). This is a learned response.

During treatment you will learn to break the association between your symptoms and reducing or stopping activity by scheduling your activities daily so that a routine is developed. Gradually, you will be able to increase the amount of daily activity until you reach a normal level. This works by gradually reversing the learned response which has been reinforced over and over again. At first symptoms are likely to get worse rather than better, but in time they will reduce, and then disappear altogether.

Assessing your problem

Do not underestimate the complexity of your fatigue problem. It is first necessary to become aware of the factors that influence it. One tried-and-tested method for assessing similar problems, such as chronic pain, involves looking at how your thoughts and actions or behaviour influence your symptoms.

First, draw a triangle like the one below, and write down the symptoms you experience. Next to each symptom write down what you do in response to the symptoms, and your thoughts. Notice how changes in one area lead to changes in another. Changing your behaviour will bring about changes in your fatigue and, ultimately, how you think.

To build up an accurate picture of your problem and how much it affects your life you must carry out a self-assessment. This involves writing down in detail your symptoms, the restrictions they place on your life, and some of the factors you think may have contributed to either the onset or continuation of your fatigue. This may

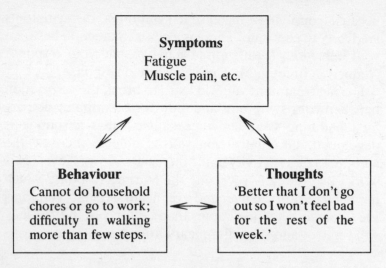

seem rather tedious, but the process itself will help you to feel you are doing something positive.

Listed below is a set of questions to guide you in your self-assessment. For the sake of clarity the questions are divided into four groups. Answer them according to how you felt over the last month.

Self-assessment questionnaire

Symptoms
- Do you feel weak?
- Sleepy or drowsy?
- Do your muscles hurt when resting?
- After exercise?
- Do you have a range of symptoms which seem unexplainable?

Thoughts
- Do you worry about doing too much?
- About the consequences of overdoing it?

- Do you have difficulty concentrating?
- Do you find it difficult to find the correct word'?
- Do you have problems with your memory?

Behaviour

- Are you able to go to work?
- To carry out light household chores?
- To do heavier jobs, such as gardening?
- Is your social life restricted in any way?
- Are your close relationships affected by your problem?
- Do you have difficulty starting things?
- How would you like your life to change?

Miscellaneous

- When did your fatigue start?
- How long has it been a significant problem for you?
- What percentage of the time do you feel tired?
- What do you think are the causes of your fatigue?
- Are you having trouble with your sleep – either sleeping too much or not sleeping enough?
- Do you feel depressed or low at times?

The purpose of this exercise is to help you to think about how your fatigue problem fits in with a typical picture of someone who has chronic fatigue. It will also help you to plan your own treatment. It is vital to see how your problem interacts with other areas of your work, home and social life. The next set of questions should give you some idea of how these areas interfere with your energy levels:

- Are you satisfied with your relationship?
- Do you get enough emotional support from your partner?

- Can you express yourself openly within the relationship?
- Do you have any financial worries?
- Are you worried about your children in any way?
- Do you feel you have enough challenges in your life?
- Overall, are you happy in your work?
- What things in your life would you like to change?

Self-monitoring

Like many people with fatigue, you may have tried to keep busy in spite of your exhaustion, but find you have a miserable time juggling what you can do in response to your symptoms. It is useful to keep a diary to build up an accurate picture of your fatigue in relation to how much you do, linking levels of activity with levels of fatigue.

Your self-monitoring record will show you how you are spending your time, and will make you aware of any inconsistencies in your activity levels, which may be contributing to your problem. In addition, it will show you how your fatigue levels vary throughout the day. You should take special note of how much time you spend enjoying yourself, and how much time you have for relaxing.

Some problems you might encounter with self-monitoring include the following:

Thinking you are doing nothing: watching television or reading are activities. Sitting on your bed resting is doing something, as is resting in a chair day-dreaming. *You are never doing nothing*. It is helpful to record such things even if they seem trivial.

Delaying writing things down: it is important to write down what you are doing and how tired you feel as you go along. If you do not you will forget very quickly.

Not having time to write things down: if you find you do not have time to keep a diary of your daily activities, it may mean you are doing too much. Stop and think about how much you really are enjoying life. Are there activities that could be cut out or reduced to give you some time for relaxing?

Self-monitoring activity record sheet

Write down what you are doing every hour of the day, however trivial it might seem. At the same time record how fatigued you feel every two to four hours on a 0–8 scale.

Fatigue rating –

0	1	2	3	4	5	6	7	8
not at all		slightly		moderately			severely	

Is there a pattern?

Looking over your weekly diary you may find you alter your plans according to either how fatigued you think you may become, or how fatigued you are at the time. When you come to planning what you do more consistently the record will help you to start at an achievable level.

You may discover that your life is somewhat hectic. Instead of reducing levels of activity in order to control your fatigue, you fill every minute of the day either with work or social and leisure activities. You may find you have little or no time for relaxing. As well, if you are under a lot of stress at the moment you may feel more tired than usual. Remember, stress is one of the main causes of tiredness.

Below is an example of a sheet completed by someone who is fatigued, but still managing to do quite a lot:

Date	Time	Fatigue rating	Activity (hourly)
3 July	8 am	6	Getting up and dressed/ breakfast
	9am		Housework
	10 am	5	Shopping
	11 am		Reading/ sitting
	noon	6	Preparing lunch
	1 pm		Resting
	2 pm	2	Resting
	3 pm		Resting
	4 pm	2	Reading

Opposite is an example of a weekly activity schedule which you can photocopy and use for your self-monitoring sheet.

Weekly activity schedule

Write down what you are doing every hour.

	Mon	Tue	Wed	Thurs	Fri	Sat	Sun
9–10							
10–11							
11–12							
12–1							
1–2							
2–3							
3–4							
4–5							
5–6							
6–7							
7–8							
8–12							

Every individual's fatigue problem is unique, so it is difficult to describe a typical case. Some of you will find you have days full of activity, and other days are spent resting because of excessive fatigue. This may not be a problem, but it is something to take special note of. Many of you will have very busy lives with little spare time, and may feel pessimistic about how you could make any changes for the better. Hopefully, whatever your level of fatigue and lifestyle, you will find something in the following chapters that will be of help.

3

Self-management

We have seen how chronic fatigue often leads to a pattern of rest and activity which is self-perpetuating, frustrating and extremely difficult to break. The next step is to begin to alter your pattern of rest and activity.

If you are doing too little

If you have chronic fatigue it is likely you are resting inefficiently and receiving little lasting benefit. The amount of rest you have may vary: the days you feel bad you may rest more, and on the days you feel good you may hardly rest at all. Perhaps you rest in response to fatigue and find it hard to get into a routine.

Resting in this way is not beneficial or refreshing. Although you probably feel you need more rest, too much rest can make you feel even more tired and lacking in energy. In addition, it impairs the quality of your sleep, reduces physical fitness, weakens the heart, reduces muscle strength and increases muscle fatigue. It can also lead to symptoms such as headaches and dizziness.

In addition to resting inefficiently, your activity levels probably tend to fluctuate. As inactivity for any length of time is frustrating, you may tend to throw yourself into things, particularly on good days. This may result in your symptoms getting worse, or a return to inactivity. The key to breaking this pattern is to plan a systematic programme of scheduled rest and activity.

Changing old patterns

The aim of CBT is not simply to be more active; if it was that simple you would not need to read this book! Rather, activity and rest need to be *consistent* rather than *symptom-dependent*. By introducing consistency you will be able to gradually increase your ability to carry out everyday activities, while slowly cutting down on excessive rest.

Goal-setting

Now that you know from your self-monitoring sheets how you are spending your time, you can plan each day in advance. Although it may be difficult at times because of regular commitments, it is important as far as possible to do the same amount of activity every day regardless of how tired you feel. This will not be possible if you are too ambitious at first, so it is crucial to begin at a level at which you think you can cope. Your goals must be realistic. Use your diary of activities to help you plan the first steps. *Be realistic.*

Write down a list of activities ranging from easy to very difficult which you think contribute to your tiredness. This list can be used along with your diary to plan the first stage of your activity scheduling. A sample list is shown below:

- doing light housework   **Easy**
- reading the paper
- lifting the shopping
- walking to the local shops
- reading a novel
- walking more than 1 mile
- socializing in the evening
- going to work
- gardening   **Very difficult**

Schedule your activity and rest by the hour. For example, write down '15 minutes' housework' rather than 'clean the house'. It is important to spread activity and exercise evenly throughout the day: rather than taking a 45-minute walk, take one walk for 15 minutes, three times a day. Your goals should be specific, and easily achievable.

The following list shows a range of goals set by someone with a severe fatigue problem. Note that the emphasis is on small achievable tasks, which are performed often:

Goals

1. Get up at 8.30 every day.
2. Walk for 10 minutes, 3 times daily (11 am, 2.30 pm, 5 pm).
3. Rest for an hour in the chair in the morning and afternoon.
4. Do not catnap during the day.
5. Do 15 minutes' housework in the morning and afternoon.
6. Go to bed at 10.00 pm.

If you start with goals that are too ambitious or unrealistic, you will surely fail. The overall aim is to carry out a very gradual approach to resuming activities. New, more difficult goals should not be set until the current ones are being carried out without difficulty. Always practise your goals for at least one week before increasing them. Practice makes perfect.

Record your goals on a daily basis in relation to your fatigue rating on a scale like the one on page 32.

Goals

1. Get up at 8.30 every day.
2. Walk for 10 minutes, 3 times daily.
3. Do 15 minutes' housework, twice daily.

Fatigue rating:

0	1	2	3	4	5	6	7	8
not at all		slightly		moderately			severely	

Date	Time began/ ended	Task	Fatigue before/ during/ after			Comments

Getting started

Getting started on a daily programme of activities is not easy; sticking to it is even more difficult. It is helpful therefore to enlist the help of your partner or a friend for support. Explain to them what you are doing and how it works. This will help you to be clear in your own mind about the approach as well.

Once you start to schedule your daily activities so that a

similar amount is done every day, it is usual to experience an initial increase in fatigue and other familiar symptoms. It is important to expect this. The increase in fatigue is usually only temporary, and in fact you may find you feel worse just before a general increase in your activity level.

There may be times when you feel like reducing your level of activity or increasing your amount of rest. You are bound to feel like this at times, but – beware! – if you succumb you will return to the same pattern that has prevented you from getting better. Rather than reducing the amount of activity, persevere with the tasks you have already chosen. In time your symptoms will subside and you will be able to move on to the next step.

On the other hand, at times you may feel so confident that you are tempted to increase your activity levels dramatically. Again, beware! You have probably tried this before and know that it usually results in a step backward rather than forward. Remember, the key to success lies in increasing your level of activity *gradually* and *consistently*.

Rest as well as activity should be built into your timetable. Do not rest when you feel tired; instead, plan to rest at set points during the day, for a certain amount of time. Start with sufficient rest to enable you to get through the day. Remember that sleeping during the day is likely to result in sleep problems at night. Try to get up and go to bed at the same times every day.

By structuring your time you will feel in control of your life again. You will also feel you are doing something that will in the long run help you with your problem. Having guidelines and structure will prevent you from sliding into a cycle of steadily worsening disability.

Writing down the day's activities will help them to seem less overwhelming. It will give you clear structure, with goals you know you can achieve. Slowly you will find yourself able to do more and your level of fatigue will start to go down.

Setbacks are bound to occur from time to time. Expect them, and as far as possible stick to your preplanned goals. Occasionally you may experience a worsening of symptoms for no apparent reason. Remember that the overall trend over weeks is what counts, not the few off-days.

Odd as it may seem, a very common fear is of getting better. Becoming aware of factors which may stand in your way can only be helpful, and may give you greater insight into what may be blocking you from change.

A common reason for feeling ambivalent about getting better is a fear of having to resume responsibilities which are no longer, or which never have been, enjoyable. For example, Jane is a single parent who previously worked as a social worker in an impoverished setting where resources were poor. Clearly, she had good reasons for not wanting to return to a situation that probably contributed to her becoming ill in the first place. During her illness she had time to re-evaluate her life and realized that she wanted to make a new start, and decided on a career change.

On the other hand, there may be a part of you that has found advantages in being fatigued. Peter, for example, was a shy man who found socializing very difficult. Not being able to join in group activities or go out with friends because he was 'too tired' provided a good reason for avoiding uncomfortable situations. To stop being tired meant Peter would have to deal with his problem of shyness.

Write down two columns headed 'Advantages' and 'Disadvantages', then list any thoughts you might have in each. It may be difficult to come up with the advantages because it is hard to see why you may want to be ill, or that you may be avoiding making an important decision or change in your life.

Maintaining progress

Your diaries are an extremely important part of treatment. It is important for you to keep a record of the goals you have set for yourself, your daily achievements, and your levels of fatigue. This helps you to keep track of where you are now, and what progress you are making. You will find that progress varies: sometimes you seem to improve in leaps and bounds, and at other times progress seems very gradual or even non-existent. The times when you feel 'stuck' and disheartened are the times that you need to be able to look back at your old diaries and see how much you really have improved.

By always having a note of your current goals you will be prevented from deviating from them. It is important at the beginning to be structured. Although it may seem rigid at times, you will slowly gain confidence at being more flexible.

As it may be impractical to fill in your diaries after every task, it is probably better to complete them twice a day at roughly the same time. If you leave them too long you will find that you will not remember what you have done or how fatigued you felt. Also, filling in your diaries can be a great motivator.

To illustrate the approach, consider the following example:

Pauline felt she had a lifelong susceptibility to developing infections. When she was 25 she had pneumonia. Although this was treated promptly, she took a long time to recover, and continued to feel fatigued for two years afterwards. She eventually made a full recovery, but developed another serious infection ten years later. Once again Pauline did not get back on her feet in the way she would have expected, and continued to feel very tired. She battled on, and as she was working full-time and had two small children, she rarely had time to rest.

Gradually her fatigue got worse until she was unable to lead a normal life. Her fatigue started to affect every aspect of her life. She had to give up work; she was no longer able to socialize like she had in the past, and found the children more and more difficult to deal with. Even light housework and cooking became difficult. Eventually Pauline was confined to bed, unable to walk more than a few steps without becoming exhausted.

Initially, she was given a diagnosis of ME by her doctor, and was told to rest as doing too much would promote the fatigue. Pauline rested completely for two weeks but felt no better. Her muscles felt like lead; heavy, achy. Every time she tried to get herself going, she felt she made the situation worse. As long as she rested she felt all right. However, she became very frustrated at not being able to do anything, and felt at a loss as to what to do.

She tried a variety of homeopathic treatments, which did not help significantly. Finally, she was seen by a specialist who diagnosed post-viral fatigue syndrome. She underwent a range of investigations which were all normal. By this time, Pauline felt very demoralized, and was mildly depressed.

She was obviously very concerned that she had something seriously wrong with her, and was afraid that the doctors may have missed something; she could not believe it was possible to feel so ill without there being an obvious cause. When the neurologist told her that all the tests were normal, she became worried that the doctor and her friends would think she was imagining the problem.

Pauline luckily had an understanding doctor, who told her she had a serious problem which needed specialist treatment. She was referred to a therapist, who helped her to adopt the treatment approaches described in this book.

She began by doing small amounts, and gradually built up what she was able to do. At first Pauline simply took short walks – a ten-minute walk every two hours. After about two months, she increased her walks to 20 minutes every two hours, and reduced the number of naps she took during the day. Pauline gradually started to do the housework again, and was soon able to do the shopping. Her confidence grew slowly. Even when she felt afraid of doing what was asked of her, she stuck with it.

By the end of treatment Pauline was able to go swimming once a week, and could cycle to the shops to do the shopping. It took many more months to reshape her life and to feel in control again, but she has now been well for several years and is working part-time as well as running the house and looking after the children.

Practical hints

There will be times when it is very difficult to keep yourself to your schedule of rest and activity. Your motivation dips and it becomes hard to be enthusiastic about the programme. Below is a list to help you keep going:

- Avoid being over-active when you are feeling good or enthusiastic. It is better to succeed in small tasks than to be disappointed by trying to do too much.

- Balance activities so that enjoyable and not-so-enjoyable activities are carried out on the same day. Start and end the day with an enjoyable activity.

- Do not be too hard on yourself. Give yourself a pat on the back when you have achieved your goals.

- Stick to the same goals for at least a week. Never increase them until you feel reasonably happy with the current ones.

- Remember that it is natural to feel anxious or worried at the thought of increasing tasks.

- At times it may be difficult to stick to your goals. Be flexible if something unexpected turns up.

- You may feel like giving up on your activity scheduling because you do not feel you have made progress, even though others may have noticed a change. Progress may seem slow at first, but it will get easier.

- Activity scheduling will be straightforward on good days. It is doing the same on bad days that is the key.

Summary

- Activity must be only gradually increased.
- Tasks must be practised regularly and consistently.
- Start with the least-difficult task and build up slowly.
- Undertake activity for short periods of time.
- Fatigue may get worse before it gets better.

If you are doing too much

The effects of not having enough time include:

- previously enjoyable tasks become a chore;
- you feel tired all the time;
- you start to feel depressed;
- you lose your temper more easily;
- your ability to concentrate is upset;
- the quality of your relationships are affected.

Never having time to rest is a modern-day complaint. Living life in the fast lane often means achievement and success. However, your body is not a machine and even machines break down. Think of a car: if it is driven fast and furiously without regular servicing it starts to go wrong. One that is taken care of, driven more cautiously and given regular servicing will last longer. You too need special care and attention if you are to remain healthy.

First, you should set aside about an hour and a half each day for yourself. This time should be strictly yours in which to do whatever you want. If you do not have time in your life now, then you must make it. Do something restful and enjoyable – put your feet up and read a book, watch TV, listen to some music.

Second, at least once a day take a rest during a busy period. Do not use this rest period for sleeping. Try to sleep for an extra hour a night.

Third, remember that pleasure and enthusiasm raise your fatigue threshold, whereas boredom and dissatisfaction lower it. Try to plan regular events which bring enjoyment into your life. This may seem impossible if you already have a very full schedule. However, by not allowing yourself any leisure time you will eventually suffer from exhaustion, sickness or depression. If you have had a recent illness, maybe it was a result of not resting enough in your everyday life.

Fourth, try to have half-an-hour's exercise at least once or twice a week, for example swimming, cycling or a brisk walk. Exercise not only increases physical fitness, but also reduces levels of fatigue, increases energy levels and improves your sense of well-being. However, do not make exercise an end in itself, something else to achieve – do it for pleasure.

Fifth, set weekly goals, which will help you to feel you

have some control over your life. Set your own limits rather than allowing others to make endless demands on you.

Sixth, lighten your workload. List all the chores you have to do in a week. Then set your priorities. If necessary, use the activity schedule to help you. Perhaps you can cut down on household chores by simply learning to live with the dirt; hoover once a fortnight instead of twice a week. Look at how you can cut down on other chores or responsibilities, which may mean lowering your standards.

This list of goals was set by someone who was doing too much and found they never had time to rest:

- leave work on time at least twice a week;
- have three evenings at home per week when working;
- go swimming once a week;
- be in bed by 11.30 pm during the week.

4
Improving your sleep

Approximately 80 per cent of people with CFS complain of sleep difficulties. If you have chronic fatigue, you may, like others, have problems with your sleep. You may find you are sleeping too much, or you are not able to sleep throughout the night. You may find that sleep is no longer refreshing.

There are many reasons for poor sleep, and not all of them will apply to you. To some degree everyone is predisposed to sleep disturbances, we have all at some time experienced sleepless nights.

Insomnia is often caused by stress or ill health. Most people resume normal sleep patterns after the triggering factor has stopped, but others continue to experience insomnia. When this happens, it is useful to examine how certain factors may be perpetuating it. The way you think and act will affect the quality and quantity of sleep you get. Strategies you may be using to alleviate the problem may be making it worse.

Arousal regulates the balance between sleep and wakefulness. It is possible that people with insomnia are in a hyper-aroused state, whereas those who sleep a lot are under-aroused. Worrying or doing vigorous exercise before going to bed, for example, would create an over-aroused state that would be incompatible with sleep. Sometimes you may notice that you are over-aroused by the fact that your heart is beating faster than usual.

The consequences of not sleeping are fatigue, irritability and an inability to perform tasks as well as usual. Symptoms of fatigue and an inability to carry out activities to your usual standard act as a reminder of how miserable your sleep was the preceding night. With time a learned helplessness develops, and your sleep problems appear uncontrollable and unpredictable.

In order to cope with insomnia, you may have developed habits, such as spending a lot of time in bed or catnapping. In the short term these strategies may help you sleep, but in the long term they become part of the problem. Daytime inactivity can lead to increased feelings of fatigue and an inability to sleep at night. It is uncommon for people with severe fatigue to take sleeping tablets. However, it is worth mentioning that although helpful in the short term, they can make the problem worse in the long run. Stimulants in tea, coffee and Coca-Cola can all cause sleep problems, as can alcohol and smoking.

The effects of lack of sleep include:

- loss of energy and drive during the day;
- decreased ability to cope with the stress of everyday life;
- decreased ability to cope with symptoms;
- feelings of depression and anxiety;
- lowering of resistance to infection;
- makes any pain worse and harder to cope with;
- reduces enjoyment and satisfaction with life.

If you are sleeping excessively, the mechanisms are slightly different. Excessive sleep is compatible with responses such as fatigue, inability to concentrate and lack of motivation. In other words, everything is slowed down.

With CFS, the more you sleep the more tired you may feel. It is not unusual for people to report sleeping for up to twelve hours or more. The fact that they are able to sleep so long but remain tired simply reinforces the belief that more sleep is needed.

Below is a model of insomnia:

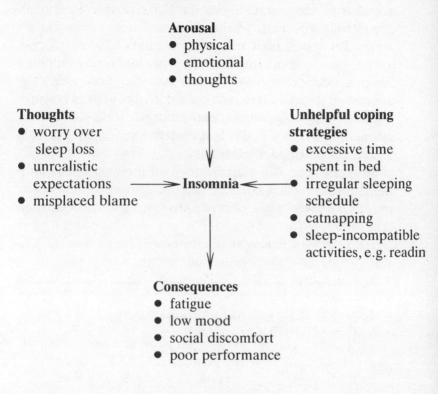

Arousal
- physical
- emotional
- thoughts

Thoughts
- worry over sleep loss
- unrealistic expectations
- misplaced blame

Insomnia

Unhelpful coping strategies
- excessive time spent in bed
- irregular sleeping schedule
- catnapping
- sleep-incompatible activities, e.g. readin

Consequences
- fatigue
- low mood
- social discomfort
- poor performance

The effects of sleeping too much include:

- loss of energy and drive when awake;
- increased need to sleep;
- decreased ability to concentrate;
- reduction of enjoyment and satisfaction with life.

Improving your sleep pattern

Many of the things I advise poor sleepers not to do are carried out by good sleepers. Many good sleepers read in bed, for example. However, it is not useful to compare yourself with a good sleeper. Instead, the aim is to get yourself moving, and change the patterns that have been interfering with your ability to have a reasonable night's sleep. This takes time and perseverance.

In order to evaluate your sleep problem it is useful to keep a sleep diary. When you get up every morning, answer all the questions. Complete the diary for two weeks initially, then calculate a 'sleep window', which is done by calculating time spent sleeping and then subtracting it from your total time spent in bed.

Maintaining a sleep diary has several purposes. First, it helps to establish a baseline of your sleep problem – you may find, for example, that you are getting more sleep than you thought. In addition, the more you understand your sleep problem the less anxious you will feel about it. You will also be able to monitor your progress over time.

Sleep diary

1 Bedtime. This is the time you go to bed and actually turn the lights off. If you go to bed at 10.45 but turn the light off at 11.15, you should write down both times in that space.

2 Length of time between turning off light and going to sleep.

3 Number of times you woke up during the night.

4 Number and length of waking-up times. Estimate the amount of time you spent awake for each awakening. If this is difficult, then estimate the amount of time you spent awake in total. This should not include the last awakening in the morning.

5 Time of last awakening. This is the time you woke up in the morning, that is, the last time you woke up.

6 Out-of-bed time. This is the time you actually got out of bed for the day.

7 Catnaps. This should include all naps, even if not intentional, for instance if you dozed off in front of the TV for 10 minutes. Make sure you specify am or pm.
8 How refreshed you feel on getting up. Use the following scale:

1	2	3	4	5
exhausted	tired	average	rather refreshed	very refreshed

9 Sleep quality. Use the following scale:

1	2	3	4	5
very restless	restless	average	sound	very sound

CBT and disturbed sleep

Sleep is susceptible to conditioning processes in the same way as our behaviour is when awake.

For those who have poor sleep, CBT has two main aims: first, to strengthen the association between sleep and bed, bedtime and bedtime surroundings, and second, to consolidate sleep over shorter periods of time spent in bed.

The first aspect of treatment seeks to change your bed time and getting up time into a shorter period spent in bed. For example, you may find that you often sleep late in the morning, take daytime naps, or spend excessive amounts of time in bed to make up for disturbed sleep. This treatment requires that you cut down the amount of time spent in bed, and establish and maintain a consistent sleep-wake cycle.

The second aspect aims at curtailing activities which interfere with the sleep process and which act as cues for

Sleep diary

Below is a sample sleep diary to help you fill in your own:

	Example	Mon	Tues	Wed	Thur	Fri	Sat	Sun
1 I went to bed at . . . o'clock and turned the lights out at . . . o'clock.	10.30 11.15							
2 After turning the lights out, I fell asleep in . . . minutes.	35 mins							
3 My sleep was interrupted . . . times.	3							
4 My sleep was interrupted for . . . minutes.	20 10 15							
5 I woke up at . . . o'clock.	7.30							
6 I got out of bed for the day at . . . o'clock.	9.00							
7 I catnapped for . . . minutes/hours in total.	20 mins							
8 When I got up this morning I felt 1 2 3 exhausted tired average . . . etc	3							
9 Overall my sleep last night was 1 2 3 very restless average restless . . . etc	2							

staying awake. The goal is to associate the bed, bed time and bedroom surroundings with relaxation, drowsiness and sleep.

Sleep restriction

Bedrest is the most common strategy used for dealing with sleep problems. If you have difficulty sleeping, you may go to bed early or stay in bed later than usual in the morning. You may also take naps during the day to catch up with lost time sleeping at night. However, too much time spent in bed, although in the short term it may alleviate some of the problems, in the long term will perpetuate them.

Sleep restriction will break this vicious circle. Use your sleep diary to estimate the amount of time you spend in bed, and to estimate the amount of time you are actually sleeping. Use your diary – if you try to guess it is likely you will underestimate the amount of time you actually spend sleeping.

For example, if you spend eight hours in bed but only six hours sleeping, then the time allowable in bed is six hours. There is no reason for staying in bed for longer than that as you are awake anyway. (Do not restrict your time spent in bed to less than five hours.)

The more you are able to restrict your time in bed the more quickly sleeplessness will become sleepiness. As the quality of your sleep improves you can increase the amount of time you spend in bed. Reassess the quality and quantity of your sleep weekly by referring to your sleep diary. Compare your sleep diary with your activity schedule. If your activity levels are low, then the amount of sleep you need will be less.

For simplicity it is easier to keep the same getting-up time but alter the time you put the light out at night. A common problem during the early stages of this approach is daytime drowsiness and fatigue. This is temporary. As you know, problems nearly always get worse before they get better. Try to think one week at a time.

Are you sleepy?

Only go to bed when you are sleepy. If you go to bed too early, it gives you time to ponder on the day's activities, think about tomorrow, and worry about not being able to sleep. Although it is likely you will be tired, do not go to bed until you are very sleepy. For example, if you have calculated that you cannot go to bed until midnight but feel sleepy at eleven o'clock, then you must fight off sleep until that time.

If you are unable to fall asleep or return to sleep within 15 minutes, get out of bed, go to another room and do something – read, listen to music, watch TV, anything but sleep. Return to bed only when you feel sleepy. Repeat this whenever you wake up during the night. This will be difficult at first, but if you persist things will get better.

Maintain a regular rising time even though you have woken several times during the night. Set the alarm clock and get out of bed at the same time every day, regardless of how you feel.

Use the bed or bedroom for sleep only. If you do not, the bedroom becomes associated with wakefulness rather than sleepiness. Do not read, eat, watch TV, work or worry in your bedroom either during the day or at night. Sex is the only exception to the rule.

Avoid daytime napping regardless of how fatigued you may feel. When you stay awake all day, you are more sleepy at night. Routine daytime naps disrupt your natural sleep-wake rhythm and interferes with night-time sleep. If at first this is impossible, a short rest on the bed for one hour may be taken early in the afternoon.

Give yourself at least an hour before bedtime to unwind.

Being active until the last minute before getting into bed can lead to feeling stimulated, which may delay sleep.

Your sleep problem will almost certainly get worse before it gets better. You may wake in the morning feeling exhausted for a while, but do not get discouraged – this is normal in the early phases of treatment; benefits will become noticeable with time and practice. Usually marked improvement occurs within two months, along with improvement in your fatigue.

Sleep is affected by a host of lifestyle and environmental factors, including diet, exercise, alcohol, noise, light and temperature.

Try to avoid stimulants such as coffee, tea, chocolate drinks, Coca-Cola and cigarettes within four to six hours of bedtime. All of these disrupt sleep in even normally good sleepers. Alcohol in excess of a couple of glasses of wine or a pint of beer should be avoided two hours before bedtime. Alcohol is a depressant, and even though it may facilitate falling to sleep, it causes awakenings later in the night.

Fit people have better-quality sleep. Very gradually build up your daytime activity, and when possible introduce exercise. Late afternoon or early evening is best. Avoid exercise three or four hours before bedtime.

Eating or drinking before bedtime should be light. A heavy meal too close to bedtime interferes with sleep. Snacks in the middle of the night should be avoided or you may become conditioned to waking when you feel hunger. Excessive drinking may lead to going to the toilet, and then problems returning to sleep.

A comfortable bed in a quiet, darkened room free from extreme temperatures and noise does not guarantee sound sleep, but it helps. Wear earplugs if noise is a problem, and an eye-shade if it's too light. An excessively soft mattress can be made firmer by putting boards underneath.

Problem-solving

If you are often kept awake at night worrying, try the following:

During the day, or at least two hours before going to bed, write down the problems which go through your head at night.

Write down the next step you need to take towards resolving each problem. Be specific.

If you wake or fail to go to sleep worrying about the problem, tell yourself that you have the matter in hand and that going over it now will not help. If a new worry occurs to you in the night, write it down or commit it to memory, in order to deal with it during your 'worry time' the next day.

You may be preoccupied with sleep itself – or lack of it – and the consequences of yet another poor night's sleep. A failure to fall asleep often leads to added efforts to control it, which in turn adds to the problem. In this case:

- Do not try to fall asleep.
- Tell yourself that sleep will come, and that relaxing in bed is almost as beneficial.
- Try to keep your eyes open. As they naturally try to close, tell yourself to resist for just another few seconds. This should tempt sleep to take over.
- If unhelpful thoughts pop into your mind, try to visualize a relaxing or pleasing scene.

Once in bed, it may be useful to practise a relaxation routine like the following.

First, concentrate on your breathing. Try to breathe deeply and slowly. Repeat silently the words 'in' and 'out' in time to your breathing. Try breathing in to the count of 'three' and out to the count of 'four'.

Next, tense and then relax your arms, neck, shoulders,

legs and stomach. Tense them for a couple of seconds, but relax for much longer. When you are able to distinguish easily between tension and relaxation, try relaxing without tensing first. Practise this at other times during the day. It is a skill which takes time, but it is worth persevering.

These will not work instantly. It can take weeks to develop new sleep habits.

If you sleep too much

It is a myth that if you sleep for, say, 12 hours, you actually need that much sleep. On the odd occasion when you are sleep-deprived it is healthy and restorative to sleep a lot. However, sleeping excessively almost every night, along with feeling fatigued the next day, is probably compounding your problem.

Cut down your sleep time gradually either by getting up earlier or going to bed later. It is best to either get up at a consistent time in the morning, or go to bed at the same time every night.

You might, for example, get up at 11 am instead of midday for one week. When you feel comfortable with this, try getting up at 10 am, then 9 am, until you are sleeping the amount of time you are happy with. Do not compensate by going to bed earlier.

This change in your sleeping pattern will initially result in your feeling more tired, but in the long run it will help you to feel more energized. The quantity of your sleep should go down, while the quality of your sleep should go up.

Remember that changing your sleep pattern will only help you to feel less tired if it is combined with other changes in your daily life.

5
Negative thinking

All of us have negative thoughts that we are unaware of. This is because negative thinking can be so habitual that it becomes automatic – it is like a reflex action. There is often a running commentary going on in the back of our minds that we are hardly aware of.

When you start your programme you may find that sometimes your thinking affects your ability to do things. For example, what you believe about yourself and your problems may stand in the way of changing. The best way of controlling and overcoming such thinking is to first identify it and then to challenge it.

This is not as easy as it sounds. Such thoughts tend to come into your mind very rapidly and unexpectedly. You probably will not be fully aware that they are occurring or influencing your behaviour because they come and go so quickly. As well, negative thinking is often logical and plausible, if not accurate. So it is not a simple matter of the thoughts being true or false.

The first step in overcoming negative thinking is to identify it. Once you can identify your thoughts easily, you can begin to examine and critically evaluate them, and then look for more helpful alternatives. Below are some examples of negative thinking:

- 'If I do the shopping today, then tomorrow I'll feel more tired.'
- 'My muscles ache today – that must mean there's something physically wrong with them.'
- 'I feel more tired than usual; I'll put off doing my planned walk today. I'll do it tomorrow.'

- 'There's no point in doing this activity scheduling. I've tried it before and it doesn't work.'
- 'I'll never get over this.'
- 'I can't possibly rest for a short time every day. I never have a minute to myself!'

Self-monitoring

Before starting your activity scheduling, try to write down your negative thoughts as soon as they occur. In addition to the negative thought, write down what precisely you are doing or thinking when the thought occurs.

You may worry about writing your thoughts down for fear of making them worse, or may feel they are trivial or silly. Remember – no thought is too trivial to write down, and before they can be controlled they have to be identified.

Below is a sample record of negative thoughts. Following that is a blank record for you to photocopy if you wish.

Record of negative thoughts

Date	Situation What I was doing	Negative thought What I was thinking (in detail)
14th May	Reading the paper.	I'll feel worse if I go out shopping; not better.
26th May	Sitting watching TV.	There must be something physically wrong – I feel tired even now, when I'm resting.

NEGATIVE THINKING

Date	Situation What I was doing	Negative thought What I was thinking (in detail)

Alternative thinking

Once you have become aware of your negative thinking, the next step is to evaluate your thoughts and to look for more helpful alternatives.

What is the evidence for and against?

There are many different ways to look at any experience. Negative thinking tends to ignore the facts. They are, after all, negative.

How else could you interpret what has happened? Get as many alternatives as you can and review the evidence for and against. Coming up with alternative thoughts does not mean you have to be positive all of the time. It simply means there are other ways of viewing the situation which may be more helpful to you. Do some of the facts contradict what you are thinking? Remember, nothing is ever all black or white. You will always be able to find evidence which supports your belief and evidence which refutes it. If you make a real effort to do this, you will begin to break the habit of thinking negatively.

What thinking errors are you making?

One feature of negative thinking is that it frequently distorts reality. Although a thought appears plausible, it may well involve thinking errors. Look for errors in your own thinking. More than one thinking error may be activated at once. Ask yourself whether you are making things worse than they are, or thinking about things in terms of black and white. Such a list is shown overleaf.

Typical thinking errors

Negative thought pattern	Description	Example
All-or-nothing thinking	Evaluating in black and white instead of shades of grey.	I'm not coping because I can't do all the things I should be able to do.
Over-generalizing	Because of one unpleasant past experience, you conclude this will occur again.	I've tried activity scheduling before. It didn't work then – why should it now?
Eliminating the positive	Dwelling on bad aspects of experiences.	So I feel good today – but most of the time I feel exhausted.
'Should' statements	Rules of living	I should always be able to cope.
Catastro-phizing	Getting things out of proportion	Any pain I have means I'm damaging my body.
Emotional reasoning	Taking a feeling as evidence of fact	I feel a failure, so I must be a failure.

Helpful alternatives

In order to challenge your negative thinking you must list all the alternative ways of looking at the situation or experience. It is essential at this stage to write all the alternative thoughts down. You can then review the evidence for and against each of them, and be in a better position to assess how accurate your original thought was. Remember, thoughts are neither true nor false.

At first you may find it almost impossible to come up with believable alternatives. This is partly because you are not used to doing it, and also because you dismiss alternatives you yourself do not believe in. It is unlikely that you will believe the alternatives at first – but do not give up. Imagine how you might advise a friend who is plagued by negative thoughts; sometimes we find it easier to look after our friends than ourselves.

What is the effect of your negative thinking?

How does thinking this way make you feel? What effect does it have on what you do? Do you modify your activity levels? Think back to the vicious circle and how thoughts can influence your behaviour.

Challenging your negative thinking

Identifying your negative thoughts takes practice. It is important that you write them down systematically every day. Next you will need to find alternatives that are more helpful to you. Overleaf are some examples of how to challenge negative thinking by finding alternatives. Try to make links between how you think and what you do. You may also be able to see how your mood is linked to the type of thoughts you are having. Keeping these diaries is essential.

Date	Negative thought	Alternative thought
	My muscles hurt because I've done too much.	My muscles hurt because I tend to do too much on one day and not enough on another.
	I can't understand why I feel so tired. I rested all day.	I feel tired because I rested all day. I need to do little, often.
	I shouldn't feel so tired; after all, other people manage to work full-time, look after children and have a busy social life.	It's normal to feel tired with so many responsibilities. I'm coping quite well.

Eventually you will be able to generate more positive ideas, but initially the negative thoughts may be too overwhelming or strong. Writing down alternative, more useful, thoughts gives them strength and power. You may not believe them at first, but in time they will become more realistic.

It is worth remembering that there is no right or wrong way of thinking. The aim of examining your thoughts more closely and generating alternative ways of thinking is to find ways of making you feel better. Everyone has negative thoughts from time to time. Eventually you should be able to control yours.

Writing down your negative thoughts and challenging them enables you to be more objective. In time your confidence will grow until you are able to challenge your negative thoughts automatically. However, practice is essential for change to occur.

Detailed record of negative thinking

Now you are practised at writing down your negative thoughts, it will help to keep even more detailed records of what you are doing and how you are feeling emotionally at the time of the negative thought. You will need to:

1 Write down the situation or event or stream of thoughts which lead to your unpleasant emotion.
2 Write down your negative automatic thought. Rate the degree to which you believe it out of a 100. Zero means you do not believe it at all. One hundred means you believe it completely. Most people score somewhere in between.
3 Specify the emotion, for example, sadness or anger, and rate its degree.
4 Write down as many alternative responses as you can think of. Rate each new belief in terms of how much you believe it.
5 Go back to the original negative thought and re-rate your belief in it. Write down how you feel now – anxious, sad – and rate it.

On page 60 is a sample table to show you how to fill in your own. Page 61 has a blank one for you to photocopy for your own use.

Situation/ Event	Automatic Thought	Emotion	Alternative Response	Outcome
Thought of going back to college.	I won't be able to keep up with the work; I'll get tired and then ill again. (85%)	Anxious (80%)	If I take one step at a time there's no reason why I shouldn't be able to cope. As long as I keep to a schedule and accept that there will be times when I get tired. (50%)	Automatic thought (40%) Emotion (45%)
Preparing to go out shopping.	I feel exhausted – I'll never feel right again. (75%)	Fed up (50%)	There's no reason why I shouldn't feel better in the future. Other people have improved using this approach.	Automatic thought (60%) Emotion (30%)
Sitting at home reading.	People don't believe I'm really ill – they think it's all in my mind. (80%)	Angry (60%)	What's important is that I know I'm ill – perhaps they don't understand and feel frustrated because there's not an obvious cause – it's a confusing illness for everybody but I'm learning to deal with it.	Automatic thought (60%) Emotion (30%)

NEGATIVE THINKING

Situation/ Event	Automatic Thought	Emotion	Alternative Response	Outcome

Challenging your negative thinking

The questions below will help you to challenge your negative thinking.

Am I confusing a thought with a fact?

Believing something to be true does not mean it is. There are often several ways of viewing a situation; rarely do we have all the facts at our disposal. Examine all the details of a situation, and use objective evidence to either back up your belief or refute it.

Am I jumping to conclusions?

This is the result of basing your thoughts on poor evidence. For example, people with chronic fatigue often feel that because something has failed in the past it will naturally fail again.

What alternative views are there?

Are you assuming that this view is the only one? How might another person look at it? Have you exaggerated, or focused on the negative?

What is the effect of my thinking?

Does it add to my feelings of low self-esteem? Am I being self-critical and expecting too much of myself? What does this do to how I feel?

What are the advantages and disadvantages?

There are always pros and cons of thinking in a particular way. However, you would feel better if you could focus on the positive rather than the negative.

Am I asking questions which have no answers?

Having regrets about the past is unproductive. There is no point in looking back – you need to look forward. Questions such as, 'Why did this have to happen to me?' or, 'Why can't I be like I used to?' serve only to make you feel demoralized. Are you sure you want to go back to where you were before? Perhaps things needed to change.

Am I thinking in black and white or all-or-nothing terms?

Typically people with CFS will have unrealistic expectations of themselves. They feel they have to do things perfectly to be satisfied. First, there is no such thing as perfection; second, rarely are people who set such high standards happy, as they are constantly striving for something else.

Am I using global words in my thinking?

Look at your negative automatic thoughts record and see whether you can spot words such as 'always/never', 'everyone/no one', 'everything/nothing'. Situations and people are rarely this extreme; it is far more likely that the appropriate word is 'sometimes'.

Am I condemning myself on the basis of a single event?

Do you condemn others on the basis of one situation? Do you make blanket judgements without considering how situations and people vary?

Am I concentrating on my weaknesses instead of my strengths?

In the face of failure or ongoing difficulties, you may be overlooking similar problems you have handled successfully in the past. Look at how you have coped with similar problems in the past, and apply the same principles in this situation.

Am I expecting myself to be perfect?

It is not always possible to get everything right all the time. People who get fatigued often have very high standards. Often the harder one tries to do things perfectly the more tired and weary one becomes. Try to lower your standards a little and see what happens.

Am I assuming I can do nothing to change my situation?

It is not unusual for people with CFS to be told that nothing can be done. Having treated many patients with severe disabling fatigue this has not been my experience.

You will find it helpful to test out your thoughts by carrying out experiments. For example, if you are concerned about doing more, then it is worth setting some goals which are achievable, carrying them out regularly and consistently, while at the same time monitoring your thoughts. You can then directly test out your beliefs, or challenge them.

Constantly questioning and evaluating our own thoughts is not something we do naturally. At first you will experience difficulty tapping into your thoughts. Do not give up when you feel discouraged. Becoming objective takes time and a lot of practice – so stick at it. Try to write down your negative thoughts every day. Question and challenge them. Then write down alternative thoughts which are more helpful to you. Beware of self-criticism: there is not a right or a wrong way of doing this. The important thing is that it will be helpful.

6

Setbacks and maintaining improvement

There will be many times when you feel discouraged. It is easy to slip back into old patterns of behaving. Expect relapses, but when they occur recognize what is happening and take some positive action.

There are times when setbacks are more likely to occur. If work becomes particularly busy or you are moving house then you may feel more stressed, and therefore more tired. Depression is closely linked to fatigue and you may find it difficult to stick to a timetable or plan when feeling low. If you do find yourself feeling more fatigued than usual, here are some hints on how to deal with it:

- Do not blame yourself. Setbacks do happen. The best way of looking at them is as a problem to be solved, rather than as a stick with which to beat yourself.

- Do not panic. Setbacks are not disastrous. Many people go through them and come out the other side.

- Remember how you changed and coped the last time. Draw on things that were helpful.

- Take some time out. Try not to feel that you have to sort everything out in one go.

In order to maintain the improvements you have made it is vital that the steps you have taken to improve your tiredness become part of your daily life. Regardless of whether you do too much, or have had to greatly reduce the amount you do it is important that you maintain an equilibrium. Days should be balanced as far as possible in terms of work, enjoyment and rest.

Help yourself!

- Exercise regularly: three times a week, half an hour of exercise. Make sure it is something you enjoy. A brisk walk in the country is enough. Do not worry if you miss a day.

- Keep a record of your negative thoughts and how they affect how you feel and what you are able to do. Challenge them – write down alternative responses.

- Try to follow a regular sleep pattern, getting up and going to bed at regular times. Try not to catnap during the day.

- Make sure your life includes enjoyable activities. Take up a new hobby if you are bored. Drop one or two responsibilities if you have too much on your plate.

- Look at your expectations of yourself: perhaps you are too demanding of yourself. Lower your expectations and give yourself credit for achievements, however small they may be.

- Eat healthily: try to eat regularly three times a day. Have a balanced diet, with lots of fruit and vegetables.

- Drink less alcohol and eliminate smoking. Both of these increase levels of fatigue.

How will you know if you are getting better?

1 By keeping a record or diary and making sure that you fill it in every day.

2 Progress may be slow at first but will speed up. Small changes are often easily dismissed or forgotten – people tend to remember failures rather than successes.

3 Look back in your diary regularly. Compare how you are now with how you were three months ago.

Index

activity *see* rest and activity
anxiety 3–4, 9, 12, 50

chronic fatigue syndrome
(*CFS*): advantages to
illness 34; assessing 21–
4; causes 3, 16–17;
identifying 1–6;
improvement and
setbacks 65–7; length of
illness 1–2, 5
cognitive behaviour
therapy (*CBT*) 18–28;
assessing problem 21–4;
disturbed sleep 45–7;
programme for those
doing too little 29–38;
programme for those
doing too much 38–40;
self-monitoring 24–8, 35

depression 3–4, 9, 11–12
doctors 3
drugs 4

emotions 1, 11–12, 16–17;
anxiety 3–4, 9, 12, 50;
depression 3–4, 9, 11–
12; effects on sleep 43;
self-assessment 22–3

family 3, 8, 13, 16, 23
food and drink 8, 11, 66;
sleep disturbance 42, 49

infectious diseases 3, 5,
10–11

mind-body problem 6–8
money worries 23
muscles 13, 20–1; painful
10–11

negative thinking 15–16,
52–64, 66; alternative
thinking 55–7;
challenging 57–9, 62–4;
self-monitoring 53–4,
59–61

perfectionism 9–10, 16
psychological illnesses 3–4,
7–9

relaxation technique 50–1
rest and activity 66; doing
too little 12–15, 16–17,
29–38; doing too much
12–15, 16–17, 38–40;
effects of 20–1;
examining patterns 18–